GET
OLD
IS WHEN...

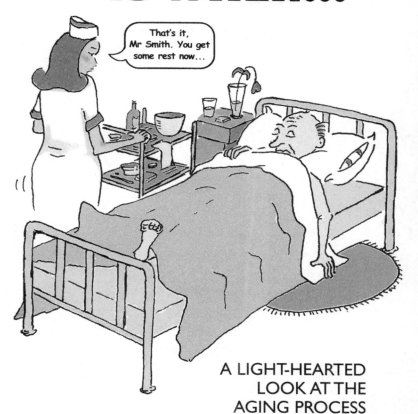

That's it, Mr Smith. You get some rest now...

A LIGHT-HEARTED
LOOK AT THE
AGING PROCESS
Illustrations by Bob Gibbs

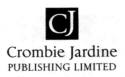

Crombie Jardine
PUBLISHING LIMITED

13 Nonsuch Walk, Cheam, Surrey, SM2 7LG
www.crombiejardine.com

Published by Crombie Jardine Publishing Limited
First edition, 2005

ISBN 1-905102-39-9

Illustrations by Bob Gibbs
Designed by www.glensaville.com
Printed & bound in the United Kingdom by
William Clowes Ltd, Beccles, Suffolk

INTRODUCTION

GETTING OLD IS WHEN....

We all know that barring accidents or illness we will live to a ripe old age and see Mother Nature run her course. As long as we keep an open mind, have a sense of humour and are not easily embarrassed, then being a senior citizen can be a lot of fun.

This book is dedicated to old age and everyone who gets there. Enjoy it and don't give a monkey's what the younger generation think: remember... their time will come!

GETTING OLD IS WHEN...

Three old pilots are strolling out to the plane.

First pilot: 'Windy, isn't it?'

Second pilot: 'No, it's Thursday!'

Third pilot: 'So am I. Let's go and get a beer.'

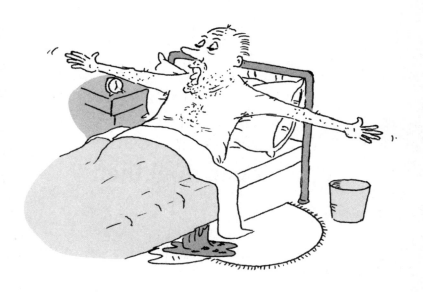

You wake at 7:00 am every
morning but crap at 6:00 am.

GETTING OLD IS WHEN...

You and your teeth
don't sleep together.

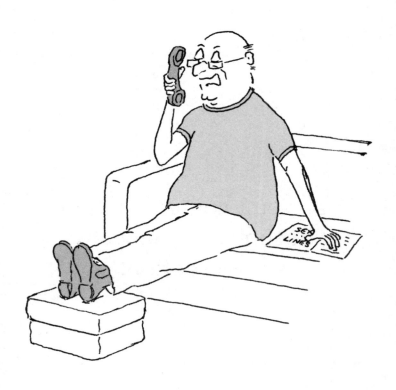

Oral Sex is just talking dirty.

GETTING OLD IS WHEN...

Your semi-annual erection
becomes an annual
semi-erection!

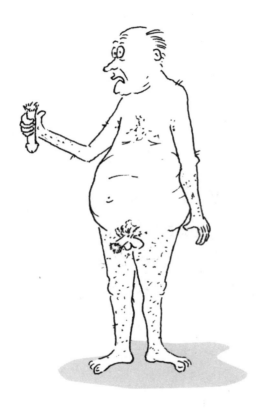

Viagra can be handy – as long as you
don't overdo it.

GETTING OLD IS WHEN...

You sink your
teeth into a
juicy sirloin – and
they stay there.

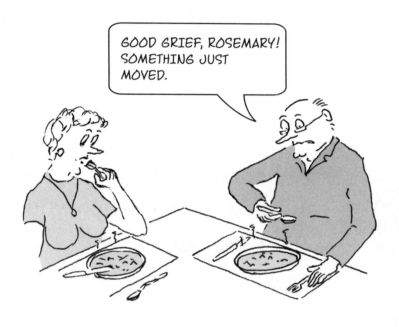

Losing your sense of taste
can be advantageous.

GETTING OLD IS WHEN...

You can't remember when your wild oats turned to All Bran.

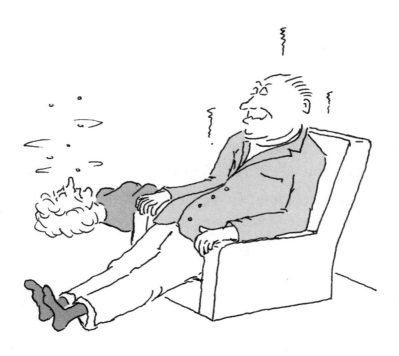

Flatulence and losing one's sense of smell can be offensive to others.

GETTING OLD IS WHEN...

'Getting a little action' means you don't need to take a laxative.

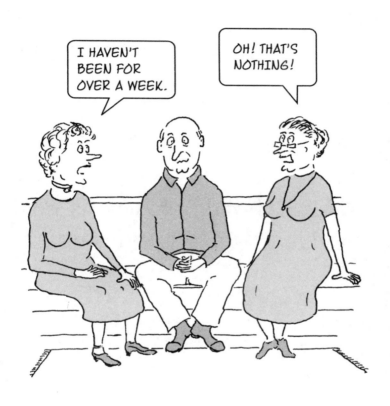

You never realized how much
you could learn about bowels.

GETTING OLD IS WHEN...

A £2.50 bottle of wine is no longer 'pretty good stuff'.

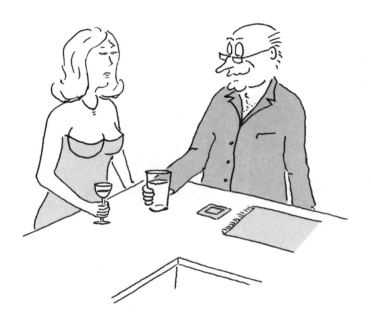

You must keep
your mind active.

GETTING OLD IS WHEN...

You have recurring
dreams about prunes.

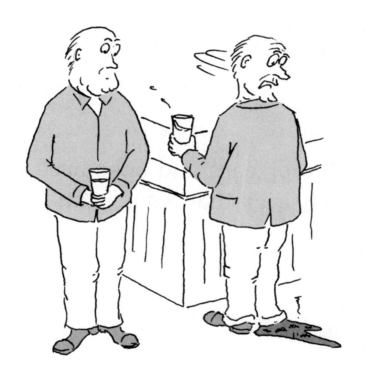

Some farts have lumps.

GETTING OLD IS WHEN...

Your ears and nose are
hairier than your head.

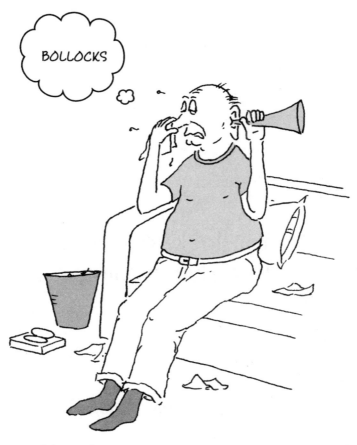

You discover the only parts
of your body *not* to stop growing
are your ears and nose... and
neither works properly.

GETTING OLD IS WHEN...

You look forward
to a dull evening.

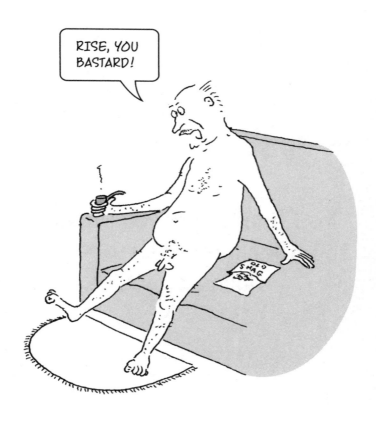

Having a shag is now
only about smoking.

GETTING OLD IS WHEN...

You finally got your head together, now your body is falling apart.

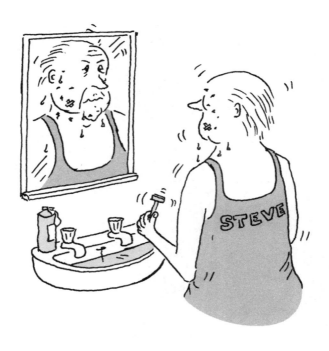

'Shakin' Stevens' has another meaning.

GETTING OLD IS WHEN...

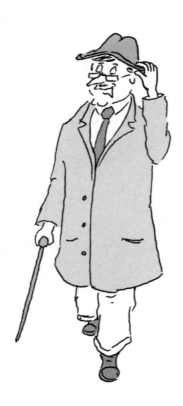

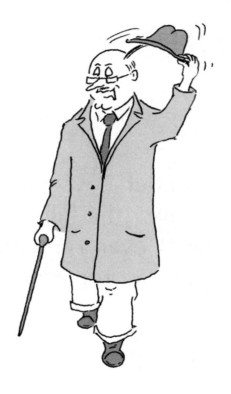

Slick has a new meaning...

GETTING OLD IS WHEN...

You wonder how you got
to be over the hill when
you don't even remember
being on top of it.

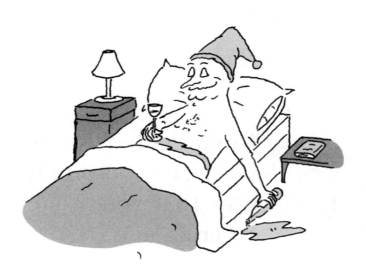

Needing a 'nightcap'
has a double meaning...

GETTING OLD IS WHEN...

You try to straighten out the wrinkles in your socks only to discover that you aren't wearing any.

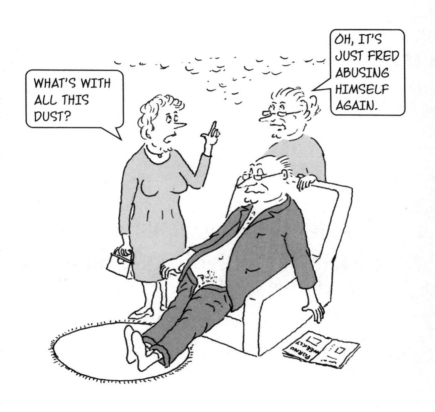

Masturbation just isn't
quite the same.

GETTING OLD IS WHEN...

Going bra-less pulls all the wrinkles out of your face.

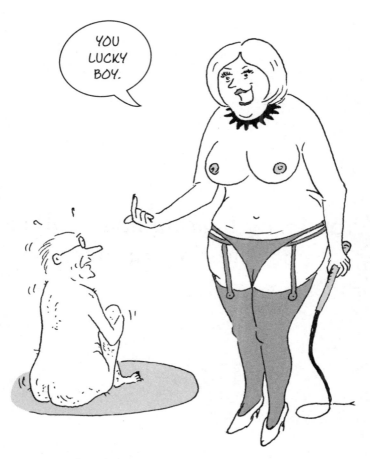

You find that you have taken on
more than you can handle.

GETTING OLD IS WHEN...

You enjoy hearing about other
people's operations.

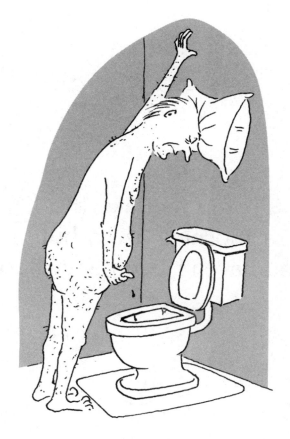

You need to get comfortable for
that quick (60-minute) leak...

GETTING OLD IS WHEN...

You feel like the
morning after, but
you haven't been anywhere.

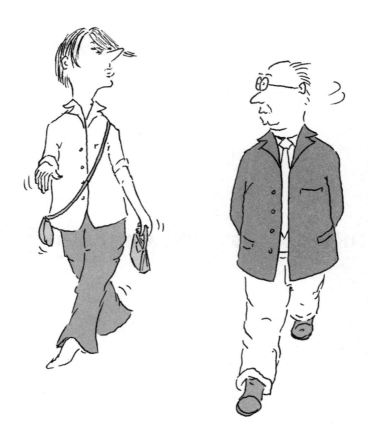

'Gay' used to mean happy...

GETTING OLD IS WHEN...

You have a party and the
neighbours don't even notice.

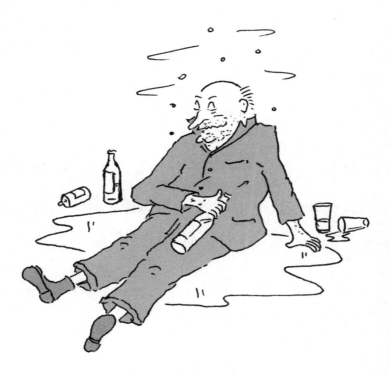

You wonder why, if drink is
so bad for you, there are so
many old drunks around.

GETTING OLD IS WHEN...

The end of your tie doesn't come anywhere near the top of your trousers.

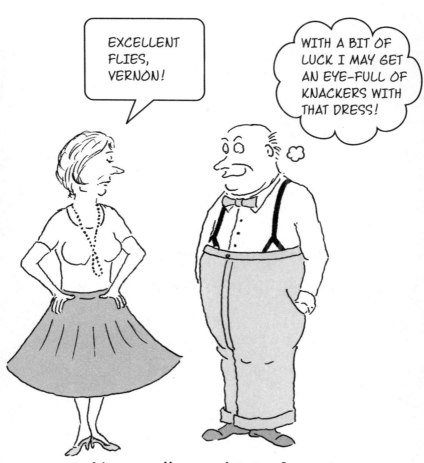

You really ought to forget
about certain fashion trends
doing the rounds.

GETTING OLD IS WHEN...

You don't remember
being absent-minded.

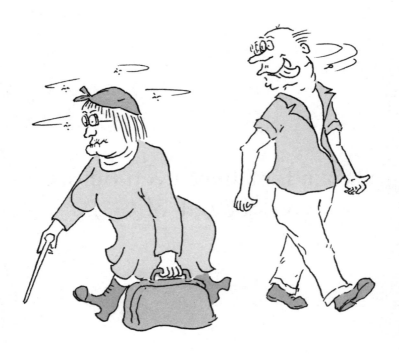

A bag lady looks attractive.

GETTING OLD IS WHEN...

Your feet hurt even before
you get out of bed.

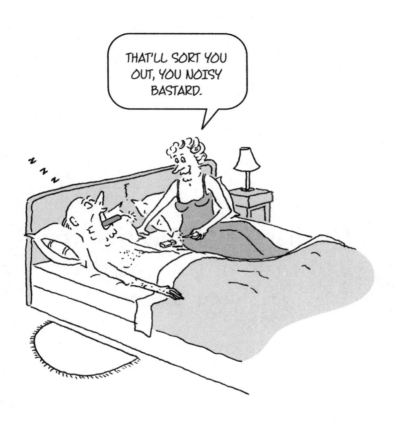

Snoring can lead to drastic action.

GETTING OLD IS WHEN...

The hardest things for you
to raise in your garden
are your knees.

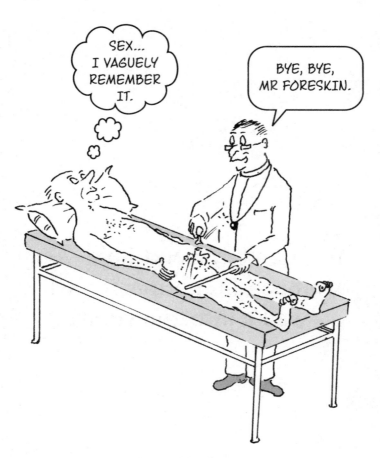

'Having it off' is now
a surgical procedure.

GETTING OLD IS WHEN...

You don't try and hold your stomach in, no matter who walks into the room.

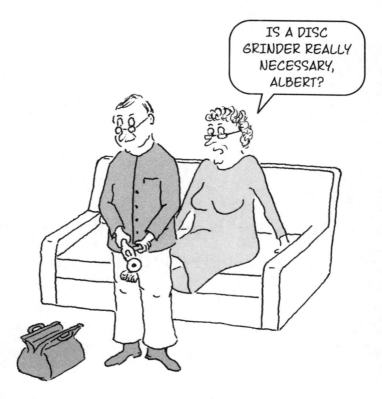

Whilst all your faculties are failing,
nails take on a life of their own...

GETTING OLD IS WHEN...

All of your favourite films have been re-released in colour.

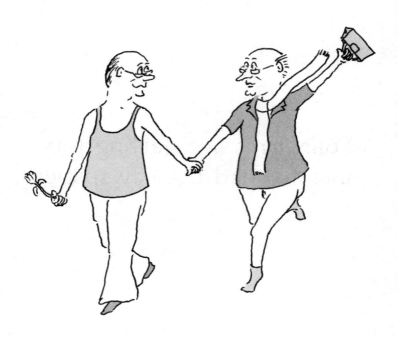

Maybe it's not the best time in life
to come out of the closet.

GETTING OLD IS WHEN...

Your arms are getting too short to read the newspaper.

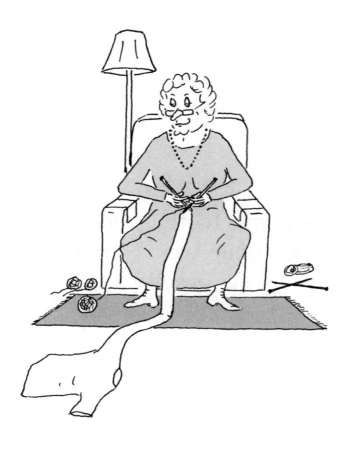

You knit endlessly
but can't remember why.

GETTING OLD IS WHEN...

You come to the conclusion
that your worst enemy
is gravity.

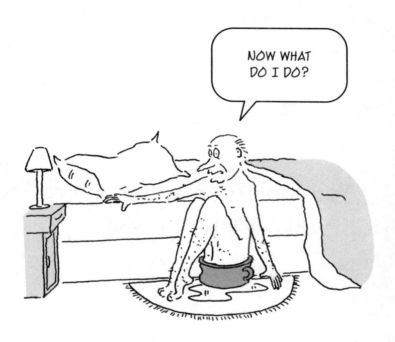

You really can get
'pissed off'
with piss pots...

GETTING OLD IS WHEN...

You look both ways before
crossing a room.

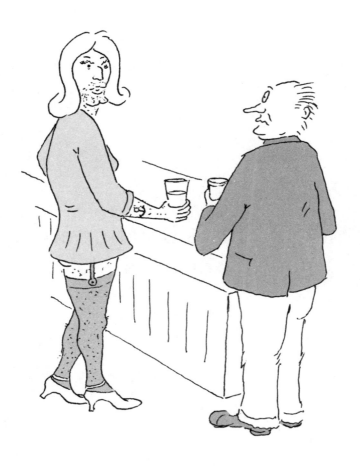

A 'tranny' used to mean a radio.

GETTING OLD IS WHEN...

You get out of breath walking
DOWN a flight of stairs.

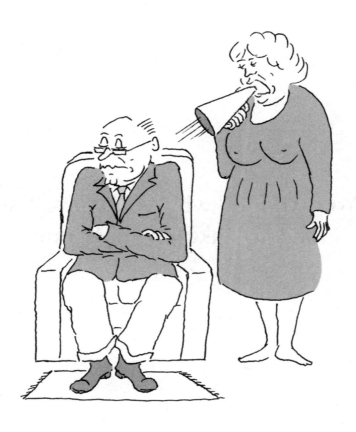

You wouldn't need a hearing aid if
everyone just stopped mumbling.

GETTING OLD IS WHEN...

You wonder why you waited so long to take up macramé.

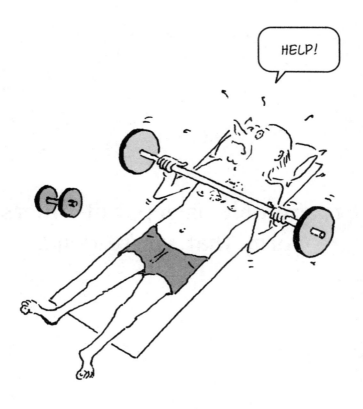

You must understand your limitations
when it comes to exercising.

GETTING OLD IS WHEN...

You're only asleep, but others worry that you're dead.

You never know when
it's time for night-nights.

GETTING OLD IS WHEN...

There is nothing left to
learn the hard way.

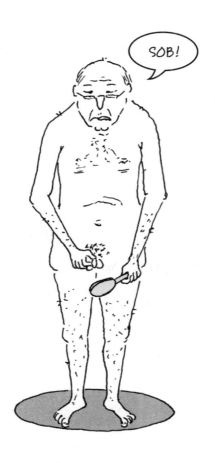

Dick used to be short for Richard,
but now it's just short...

GETTING OLD IS WHEN...

It takes a couple of
attempts before you get
over a speed bump.

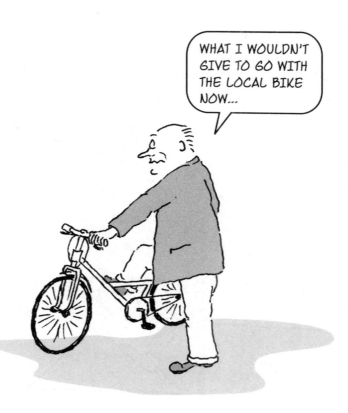

The nearest you get to a
leg-over is riding a bike.

GETTING OLD IS WHEN...

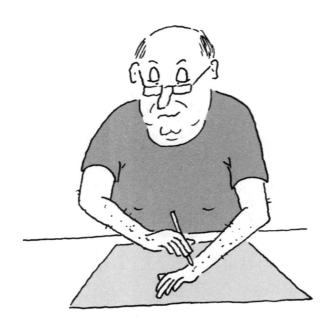

You can produce amazing drawings
by joining up your liver spots.

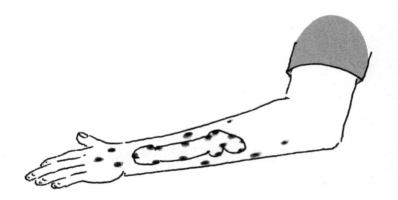

Another masterpiece...

GETTING OLD IS WHEN...

Your supply of brain cells
is finally down to a
manageable size.

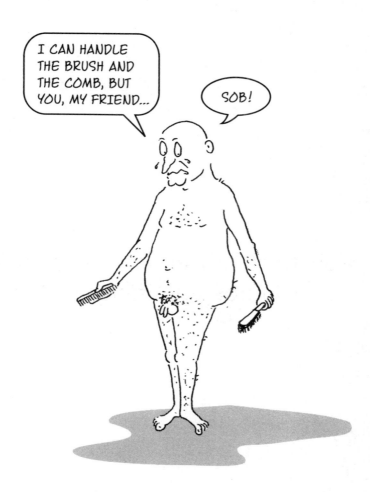

Some things become redundant.

GETTING OLD IS WHEN...

You think coffee is one of the most important things in life.

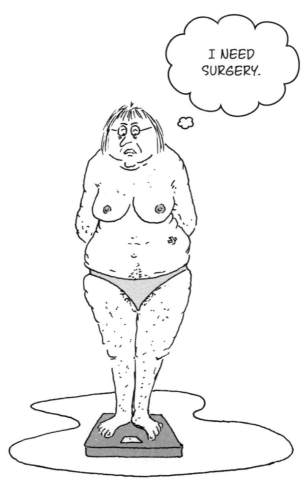

You have one of those
days... every day.

GETTING OLD IS WHEN...

Your secrets are safe with
your friends: they can't
remember them either.

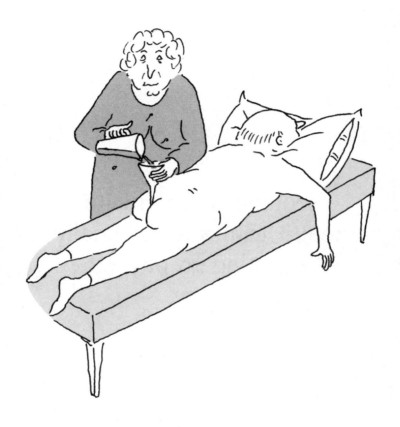

Nature needs a helping hand.

GETTING OLD IS WHEN...

Your investment in
health insurance is finally
beginning to pay off.

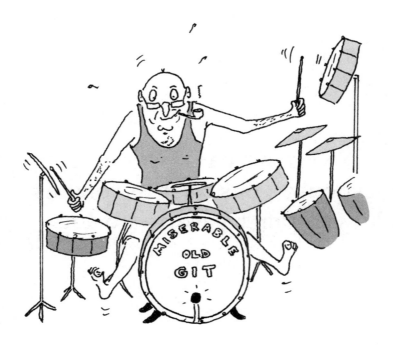

You can amuse your friends with a
quiet night in, having taken up playing
a musical instrument.

GETTING OLD IS WHEN...

You don't care where your spouse goes, just as long as you don't have to go too.

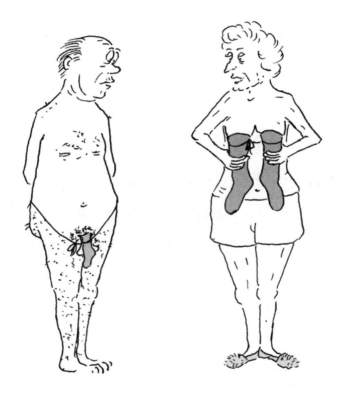

Socks become multi-functional.

GETTING OLD IS WHEN...

Your childhood toys are now museum exhibits.

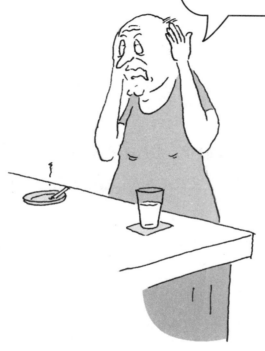

There used to be a time when ringing was the sound of either the 'phone or church bells. Now it's only ever tinnitus.

GETTING OLD IS WHEN...

Your new easy chair has more options than your car.

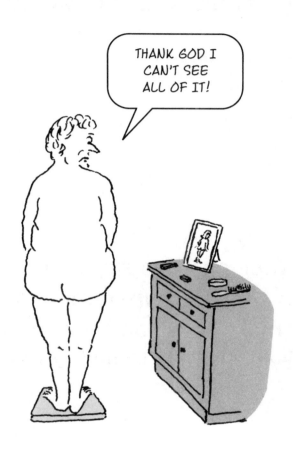

What used to be a 'tight bum'
is now a 'lard arse'.

GETTING OLD IS WHEN...

Your partner says, 'Darling,
let's go upstairs and
make love,' and you reply,
'Sweetheart, I can't do both!'

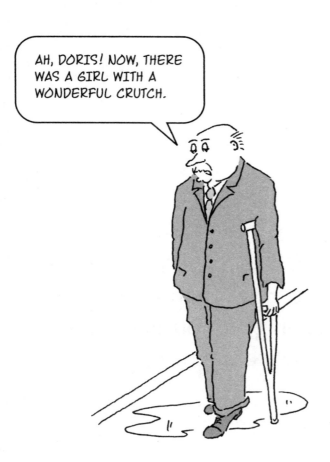

Getting to grips with a crutch used to
be an entirely different experience.

GETTING OLD IS WHEN...

You seem to have a lot more patience now than before but the reality is you just don't care anymore.

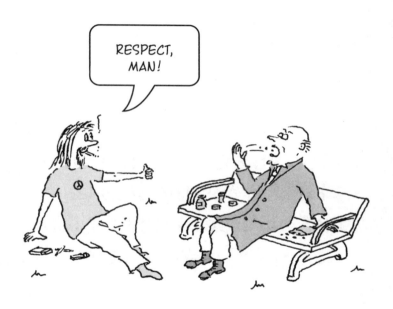

You are totally amazed by the amount of medication you have to take each day just to keep going.

GETTING OLD IS WHEN...

You spend half an hour
looking for the glasses
that have been on the top
on your head all along.

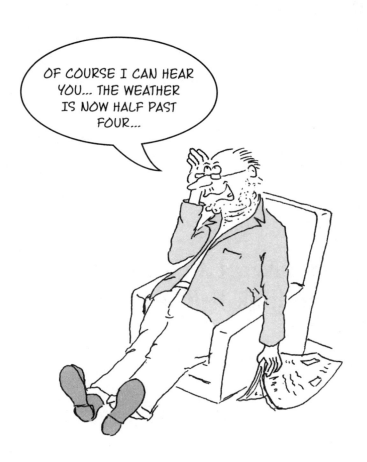

You really do need a hearing aid...

GETTING OLD IS WHEN...

It takes twice as long
to look half as good.

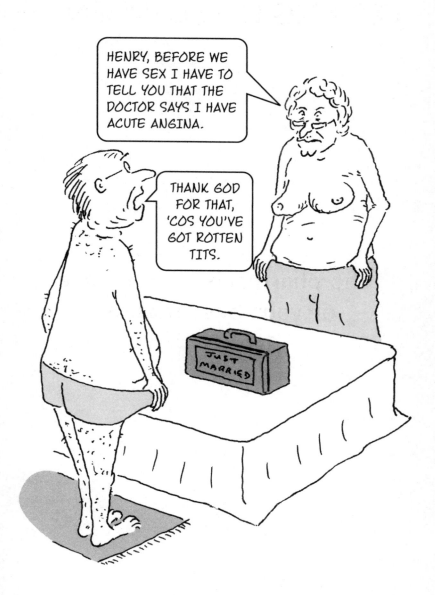

91

GETTING OLD IS WHEN...

The pharmacist is now one
of your best friends.

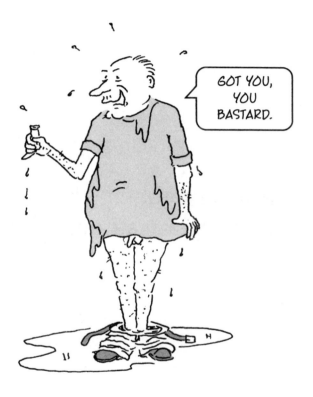

Samples can be tricky...

GETTING OLD IS WHEN...

You remember when the Dead Sea was only sick.

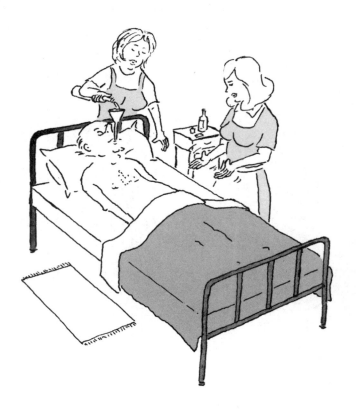

The 'clap' is now applause
for downing your medicine.

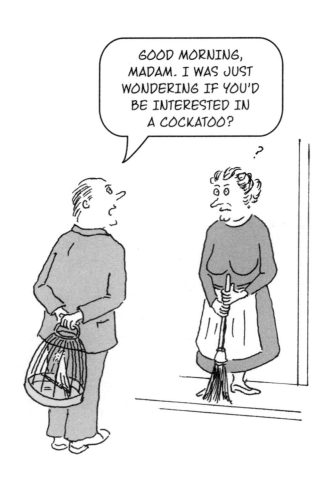

People often get the wrong
end of the stick...

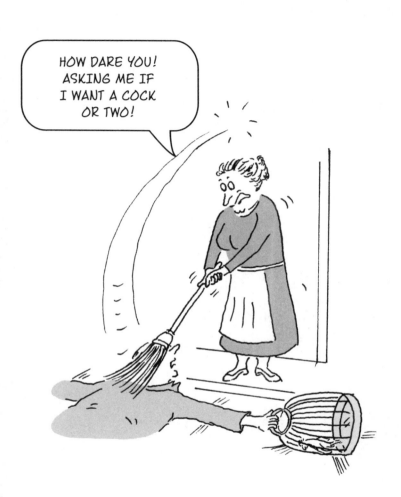

GETTING OLD IS WHEN...

Everything hurts.
What doesn't hurt,
doesn't work.

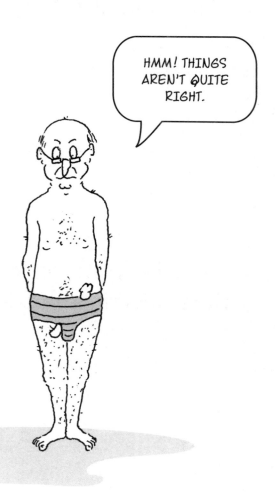

There's not a lot of room for error when putting on a truss.

GETTING OLD IS WHEN...

You keep more food
than beer in the fridge.

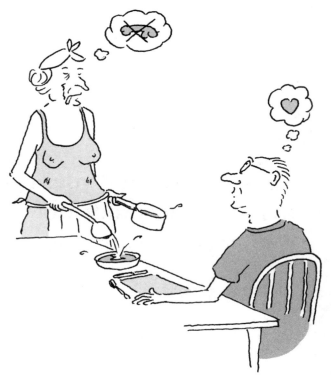

Getting your 'oats' now means
porridge for breakfast.

GETTING OLD IS WHEN...

All you want for your
birthday is to not be
reminded of your age.

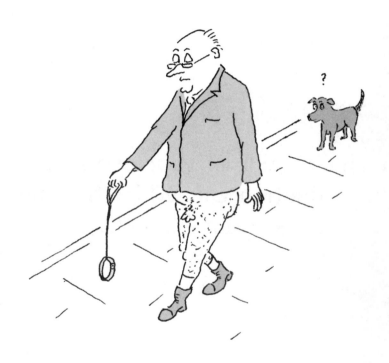

You become that bit forgetful...

GETTING OLD IS WHEN...

The twinkle in your eye is just
a reflection caused by the sun
on your bifocals.

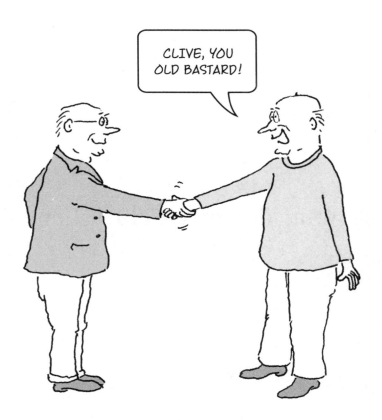

It appears that illegitimacy
procreates long life.

GETTING OLD IS WHEN...

Your idea of weight lifting
is standing up.

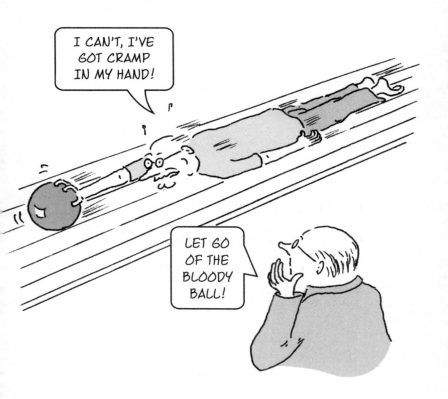

You find that some sports
are better left alone...

GETTING OLD IS WHEN...

'Getting lucky' means being
able to find your vehicle
in the car park.

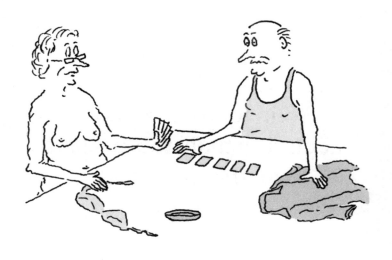

Strip poker loses its magic.

GETTING OLD IS WHEN...

Your joints are more
accurate than the evening
weather forecast.

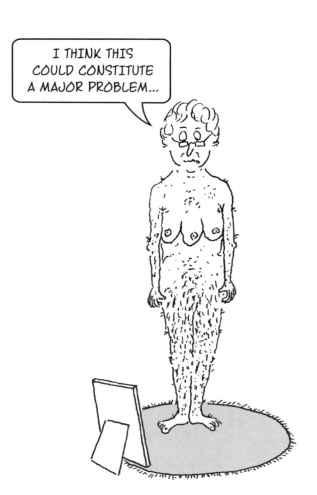

You find those drugs you've been
taking have side effects.

GETTING OLD IS WHEN...

Your back goes out
more than you do.

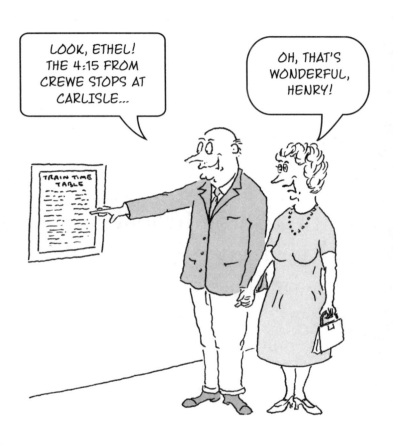

Mundane is now exciting.

GETTING OLD IS WHEN...

You're on holiday and
your energy runs out
before your money.

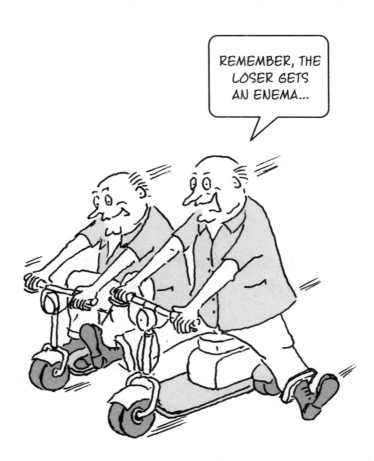

You mustn't lose that
competitive spirit.

GETTING OLD IS WHEN...

You sit in a rocking chair
but can't get it going.

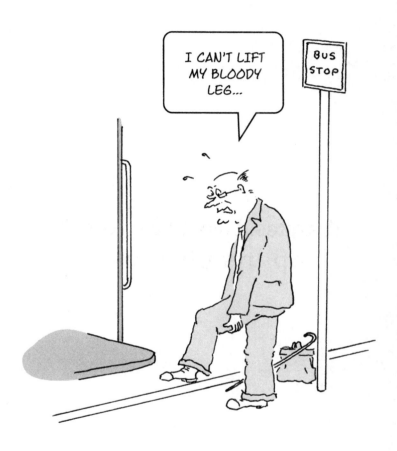

You've got a bus pass but can't use it.

GETTING OLD IS WHEN...

It takes two tries to get
up from the sofa.

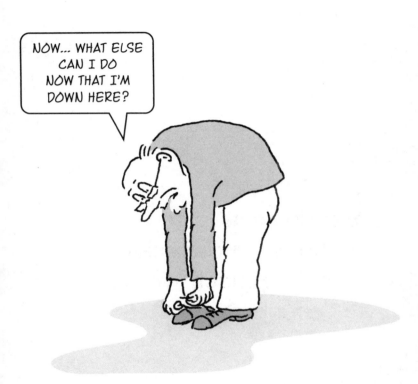

You have to seize the moment.

GETTING OLD IS WHEN...

You don't have to worry
about your eyesight
getting much worse.

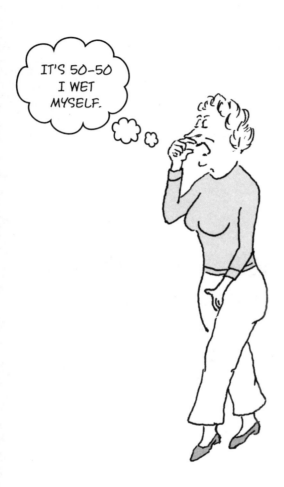

You become terrified of sneezing.

GETTING OLD IS WHEN...

It takes longer to rest than it does to get tired.

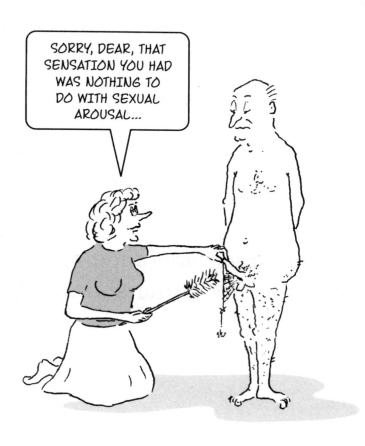

Certain bits of your body
become redundant.

GETTING OLD IS WHEN...

You start videotaping
daytime TV game shows.

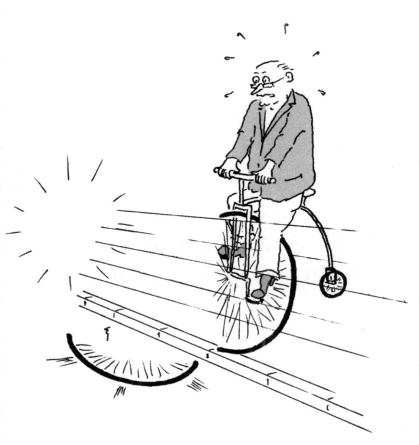

You may not be up to integrating
with today's traffic...

GETTING OLD IS WHEN...

Your idea of a night out is
sitting on the patio.

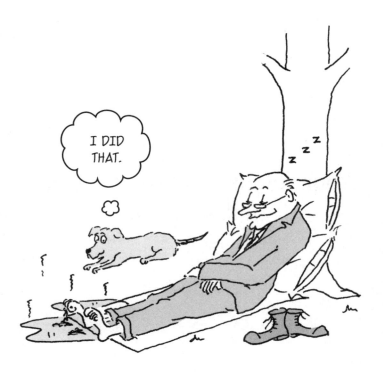

Losing your sense of smell
can have its advantages.

GETTING OLD IS WHEN...

Your knees buckle and your belt will not.

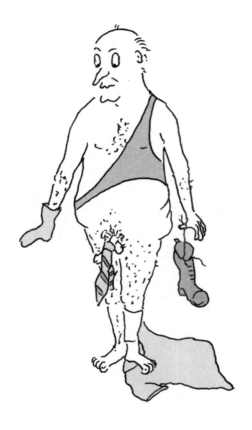

You're all fingers and thumbs
when it comes to dressing.

GETTING OLD IS WHEN...

6:00 am is when you get up,
not when you go to sleep.

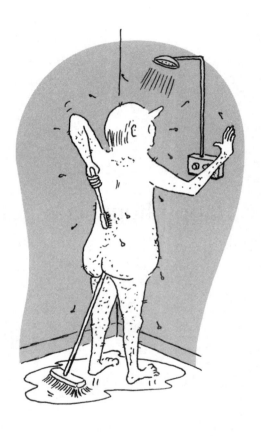

Balancing yourself upright in the
shower is an art form.

GETTING OLD IS WHEN...

'Happy hour' is a nap.

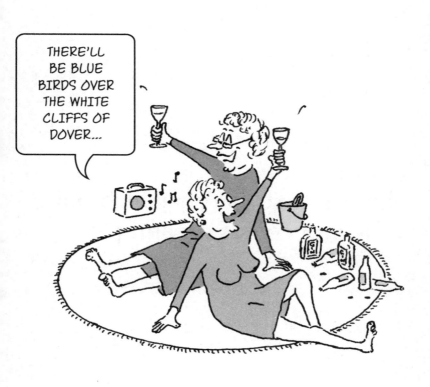

Vera is fondly remembered with gin.

GETTING OLD IS WHEN...

The car that you bought brand new becomes an antique.

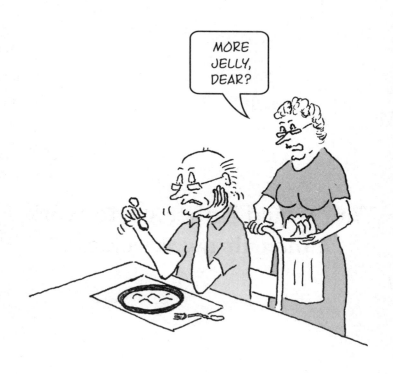

It seems that all food is tough.

GETTING OLD IS WHEN...

You would rather go to work
than throw a sickie.

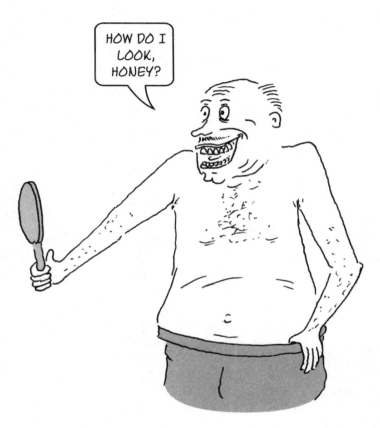

You don't want to find out
that your dentist has a wicked
sense of humour...

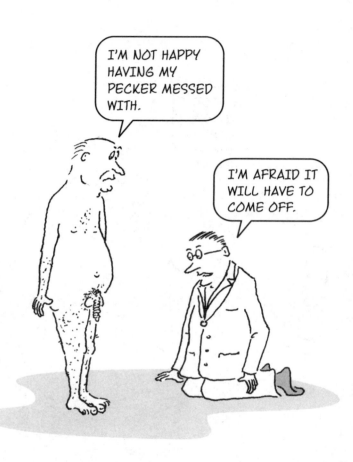

Circumcision late in life
has its problems.

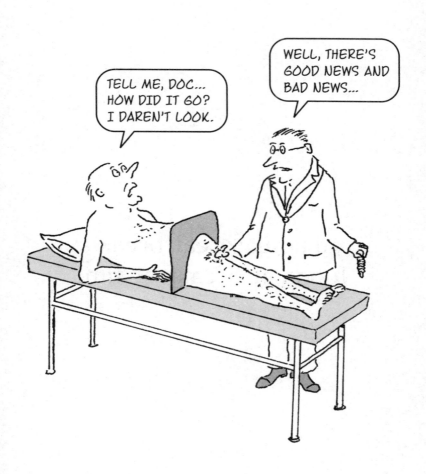

139

GETTING OLD IS WHEN...

You actually eat breakfast
foods at breakfast time.

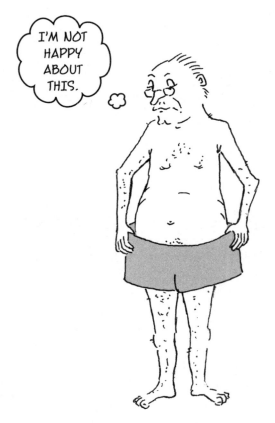

Your underpants being starched is the
nearest you're going to get to a 'stiffy'.

GETTING OLD IS WHEN...

You sing along to lift music.

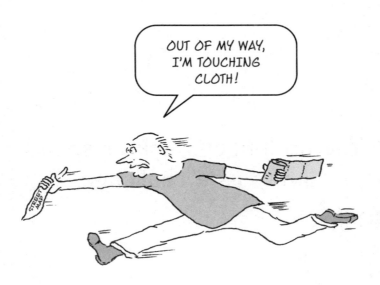

You never leave home without a
street map of all public toilets.

GETTING OLD IS WHEN...

You no longer think of speed
limits as a challenge.

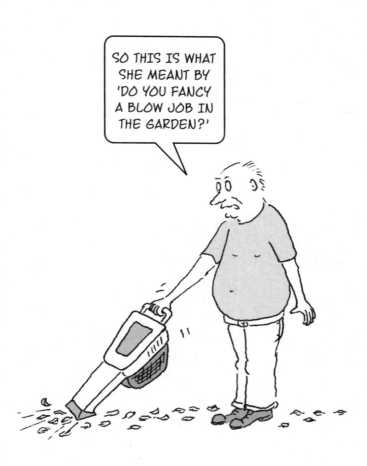

You are easily lured into doing
things due to confusion...

GETTING OLD IS WHEN...

Your children are beginning
to look middle-aged.

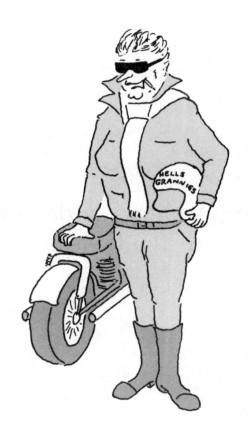

You can rediscover yourself.

GETTING OLD IS WHEN...

You take a metal detector
to the beach.

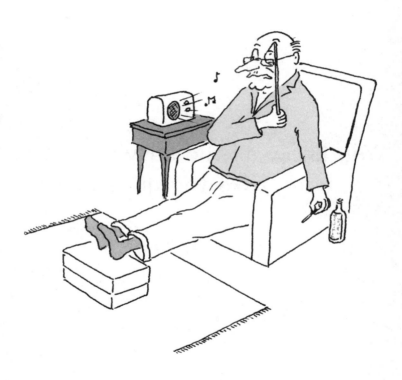

You don't sleep at night but stay
awake during the day.

GETTING OLD IS WHEN...

You know all the answers, but nobody asks the questions.

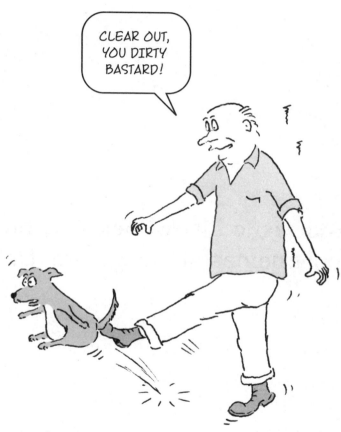

You should always have a pet to hand
in case you fart in company.

GETTING OLD IS WHEN...

Your little black book contains only names starting with 'Dr.'

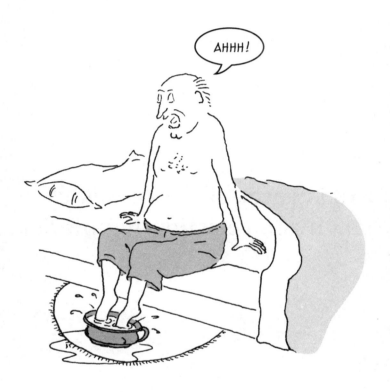

That essential piss pot has to
be kept well under the bed.

GETTING OLD IS WHEN...

You regret all those mistakes you made resisting temptation.

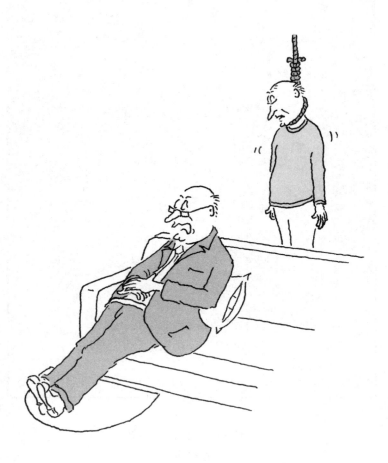

You develop a natural ability to
bore the shit out of people...

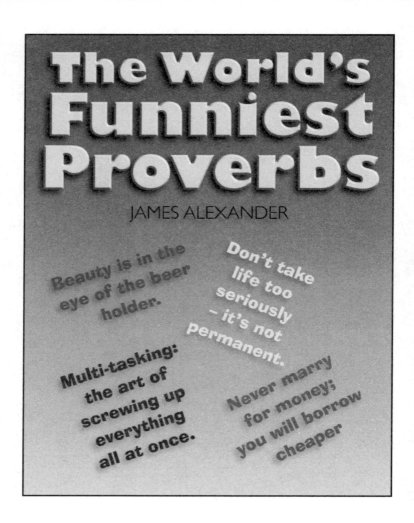

The World's
Funniest
Proverbs

JAMES ALEXANDER

Beauty is in the eye of the beer holder.

Don't take life too seriously – it's not permanent.

Multi-tasking: the art of screwing up everything all at once.

Never marry for money; you will borrow cheaper

ISBN 1-905102-02-X
£3.99

The World's Funniest Laws

JAMES ALEXANDER

In Arizona you can go to prison for 25 years for cutting down a cactus!

Do not say "oh boy" in Jonesborough, Georgia. It's illegal!

On Sundays in Florida, widows must not go parachuting!

It is against the law to take a lion to the cinema in Baltimore!

ISBN 1-905102-10-0
£4.99

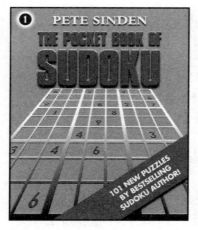

ISBN 1-905102-43-7
£2.99

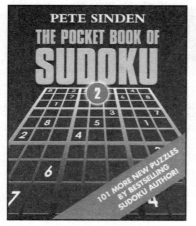

ISBN 1-905102-45-3
£2.99

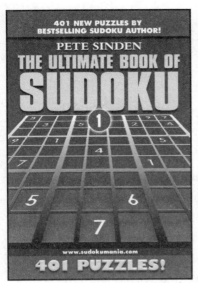

ISBN 1-905102-42-9
£4.99

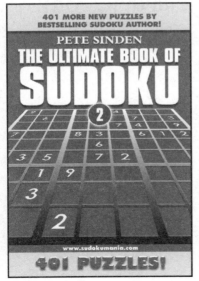

ISBN 1-905102-44-5
£4.99

All Crombie Jardine books are available from your
High Street bookshops, Amazon,
Littlehampton Book Services, or Bookpost
(P.O.Box 29, Douglas, Isle of Man, IM99 1BQ.
tel: 01624 677 237, email: bookshop@enterprise.net.
Free postage and packing within the UK).

www.crombiejardine.com